Your WEIG won't be **EASY**, but it will be **WORTH IT.**

Use this journal to help you every step of the way.

- FOOD JOURNAL
- HABIT TRACKER
- EXERCISE LOG
- MEAL PLANNER
- LIFESTYLE CHANGE PROMPTS
JOURNAL PAGES
AND MORE!

WEIGHT TRACKER

Write your goal and colour in each milestone!

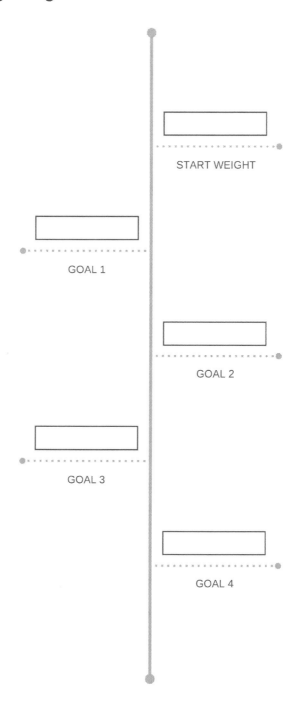

START WEIGHT

GOAL 1

GOAL 2

GOAL 3

GOAL 4

WEIGHT TRACKER

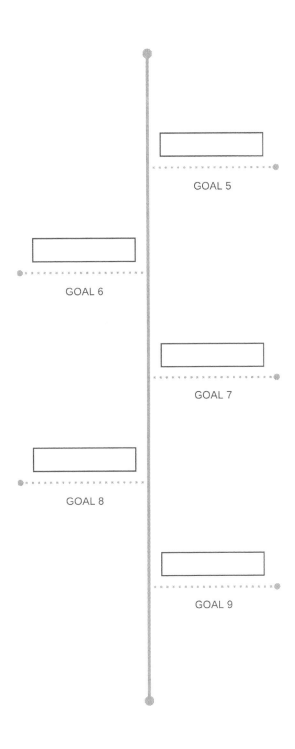

GOAL 5

GOAL 6

GOAL 7

GOAL 8

GOAL 9

FOOD	QUANTITY	CALORIES/VALUE
		TOTAL

HABIT TRACKER

HABIT   FREQUENCY

FOOD	QUANTITY	CALORIES/VALUE
		TOTAL

FOOD	QUANTITY	CALORIES/VALUE
		TOTAL

FOOD	QUANTITY	CALORIES/VALUE
		TOTAL

EXERCISE LOG

DATE	ACTIVITY	DURATION

MOOD TRACKER

GIVE A COLOUR TO EACH MOOD AND
COLOUR IN YOUR MOOD AT THE END
OF EACH DAY TO KEEP TRACK

☐ HAPPY   ☐ NEUTRAL

☐ STRESSED   ☐ FOCUSED

☐ SAD   ☐ CALM

M   T   W   T   F   S   S

HABIT TRACKER

HABIT   FREQUENCY

FOOD	QUANTITY	CALORIES/VALUE
		TOTAL

FOOD	QUANTITY	CALORIES/VALUE
		TOTAL

FOOD	QUANTITY	CALORIES/VALUE
		TOTAL

FOOD	QUANTITY	CALORIES/VALUE
		TOTAL

FOOD	QUANTITY	CALORIES/VALUE
		TOTAL

FOOD	QUANTITY	CALORIES/VALUE
		TOTAL

HABIT TRACKER

HABIT   FREQUENCY

MOOD TRACKER

GIVE A COLOUR TO EACH MOOD AND
COLOUR IN YOUR MOOD AT THE END
OF EACH DAY TO KEEP TRACK

☐ HAPPY   ☐ NEUTRAL

☐ STRESSED   ☐ FOCUSED

☐ SAD   ☐ CALM

M   T   W   T   F   S   S

EXERCISE LOG

DATE	ACTIVITY	DURATION

FOOD	QUANTITY	CALORIES/VALUE
		TOTAL

FOOD	QUANTITY	CALORIES/VALUE
		TOTAL

FOOD	QUANTITY	CALORIES/VALUE
		TOTAL

FOOD	QUANTITY	CALORIES/VALUE
		TOTAL

FOOD	QUANTITY	CALORIES/VALUE
		TOTAL

FOOD	QUANTITY	CALORIES/VALUE
		TOTAL

FOOD	QUANTITY	CALORIES/VALUE
		TOTAL

MOOD TRACKER

GIVE A COLOUR TO EACH MOOD AND
COLOUR IN YOUR MOOD AT THE END
OF EACH DAY TO KEEP TRACK

- HAPPY
- STRESSED
- SAD

- NEUTRAL
- FOCUSED
- CALM

M T W T F S S

EXERCISE LOG

DATE	ACTIVITY	DURATION

HABIT TRACKER

HABIT   FREQUENCY

MEAL PLANNER

BREAKFAST

LUNCH

DINNER

SNACKS

MEAL PLANNER

BREAKFAST

LUNCH

DINNER

SNACKS

MEAL PLANNER

BREAKFAST

LUNCH

DINNER

SNACKS

MEAL PLANNER

BREAKFAST

LUNCH

DINNER

SNACKS

FOOD	QUANTITY	CALORIES/VALUE
		TOTAL

HABIT TRACKER

HABIT   FREQUENCY

FOOD	QUANTITY	CALORIES/VALUE
		TOTAL

FOOD	QUANTITY	CALORIES/VALUE
		TOTAL

EXERCISE LOG

DATE	ACTIVITY	DURATION

MOOD TRACKER

GIVE A COLOUR TO EACH MOOD AND
COLOUR IN YOUR MOOD AT THE END
OF EACH DAY TO KEEP TRACK

☐ HAPPY   ☐ NEUTRAL

☐ STRESSED   ☐ FOCUSED

☐ SAD   ☐ CALM

M T W T F S S

HABIT TRACKER

HABIT　　　　　　　FREQUENCY

FOOD	QUANTITY	CALORIES/VALUE
		TOTAL

FOOD	QUANTITY	CALORIES/VALUE
		TOTAL

FOOD	QUANTITY	CALORIES/VALUE
		TOTAL

FOOD	QUANTITY	CALORIES/VALUE
		TOTAL

FOOD	QUANTITY	CALORIES/VALUE
		TOTAL

FOOD	QUANTITY	CALORIES/VALUE
		TOTAL

HABIT TRACKER

HABIT

FREQUENCY

MOOD TRACKER

GIVE A COLOUR TO EACH MOOD AND
COLOUR IN YOUR MOOD AT THE END
OF EACH DAY TO KEEP TRACK

HAPPY

STRESSED

SAD

NEUTRAL

FOCUSED

CALM

M   T   W   T   F   S   S

EXERCISE LOG

DATE	ACTIVITY	DURATION

FOOD	QUANTITY	CALORIES/VALUE
		TOTAL

FOOD	QUANTITY	CALORIES/VALUE
		TOTAL

FOOD	QUANTITY	CALORIES/VALUE
		TOTAL

FOOD	QUANTITY	CALORIES/VALUE
		TOTAL

FOOD	QUANTITY	CALORIES/VALUE
		TOTAL

FOOD	QUANTITY	CALORIES/VALUE
		TOTAL

FOOD	QUANTITY	CALORIES/VALUE
		TOTAL

MOOD TRACKER

GIVE A COLOUR TO EACH MOOD AND
COLOUR IN YOUR MOOD AT THE END
OF EACH DAY TO KEEP TRACK

☐ HAPPY   ☐ NEUTRAL

☐ STRESSED   ☐ FOCUSED

☐ SAD   ☐ CALM

M   T   W   T   F   S   S

EXERCISE LOG

DATE	ACTIVITY	DURATION

HABIT TRACKER

HABIT   FREQUENCY

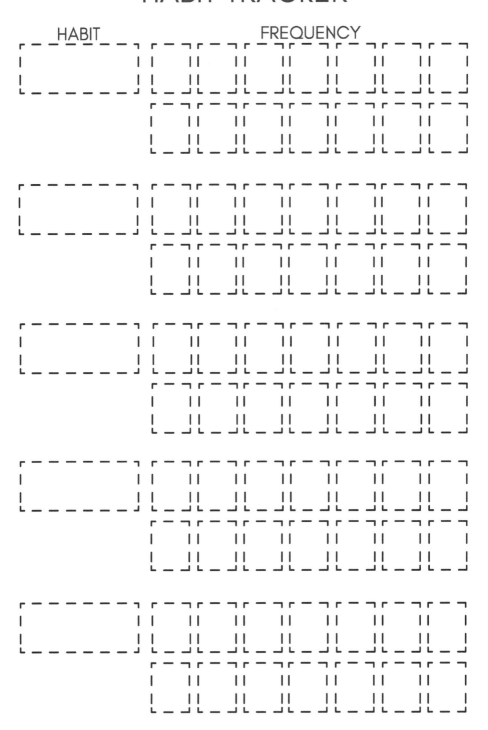

MEAL PLANNER

BREAKFAST

LUNCH

DINNER

SNACKS

MEAL PLANNER

BREAKFAST

LUNCH

DINNER

SNACKS

MEAL PLANNER

BREAKFAST

LUNCH

DINNER

SNACKS

MEAL PLANNER

BREAKFAST

LUNCH

DINNER

SNACKS

FOOD	QUANTITY	CALORIES/VALUE
		TOTAL

HABIT TRACKER

HABIT   FREQUENCY

FOOD	QUANTITY	CALORIES/VALUE
		TOTAL

FOOD	QUANTITY	CALORIES/VALUE
		TOTAL

EXERCISE LOG

DATE	ACTIVITY	DURATION

MOOD TRACKER

GIVE A COLOUR TO EACH MOOD AND
COLOUR IN YOUR MOOD AT THE END
OF EACH DAY TO KEEP TRACK

HAPPY

STRESSED

SAD

NEUTRAL

FOCUSED

CALM

M T W T F S S

HABIT TRACKER

HABIT   FREQUENCY

FOOD	QUANTITY	CALORIES/VALUE
		TOTAL

FOOD	QUANTITY	CALORIES/VALUE
		TOTAL

FOOD	QUANTITY	CALORIES/VALUE
		TOTAL

FOOD	QUANTITY	CALORIES/VALUE
		TOTAL

FOOD	QUANTITY	CALORIES/VALUE
		TOTAL

FOOD	QUANTITY	CALORIES/VALUE
		TOTAL

HABIT TRACKER

HABIT   FREQUENCY

MOOD TRACKER

GIVE A COLOUR TO EACH MOOD AND
COLOUR IN YOUR MOOD AT THE END
OF EACH DAY TO KEEP TRACK

HAPPY

STRESSED

SAD

NEUTRAL

FOCUSED

CALM

M   T   W   T   F   S   S

EXERCISE LOG

DATE	ACTIVITY	DURATION

FOOD	QUANTITY	CALORIES/VALUE
		TOTAL

FOOD	QUANTITY	CALORIES/VALUE
		TOTAL

FOOD	QUANTITY	CALORIES/VALUE
		TOTAL

FOOD	QUANTITY	CALORIES/VALUE
		TOTAL

FOOD	QUANTITY	CALORIES/VALUE
		TOTAL

FOOD	QUANTITY	CALORIES/VALUE
		TOTAL

FOOD	QUANTITY	CALORIES/VALUE
		TOTAL

MOOD TRACKER

GIVE A COLOUR TO EACH MOOD AND
COLOUR IN YOUR MOOD AT THE END
OF EACH DAY TO KEEP TRACK

	HAPPY		NEUTRAL
	STRESSED		FOCUSED
	SAD		CALM

M   T   W   T   F   S   S

EXERCISE LOG

DATE	ACTIVITY	DURATION

HABIT TRACKER

HABIT   FREQUENCY

MEAL PLANNER

BREAKFAST

LUNCH

DINNER

SNACKS

MEAL PLANNER

BREAKFAST

LUNCH

DINNER

SNACKS

MEAL PLANNER

BREAKFAST

LUNCH

DINNER

SNACKS

MEAL PLANNER

BREAKFAST

LUNCH

DINNER

SNACKS

FOOD	QUANTITY	CALORIES/VALUE
		TOTAL

HABIT TRACKER

HABIT

FREQUENCY

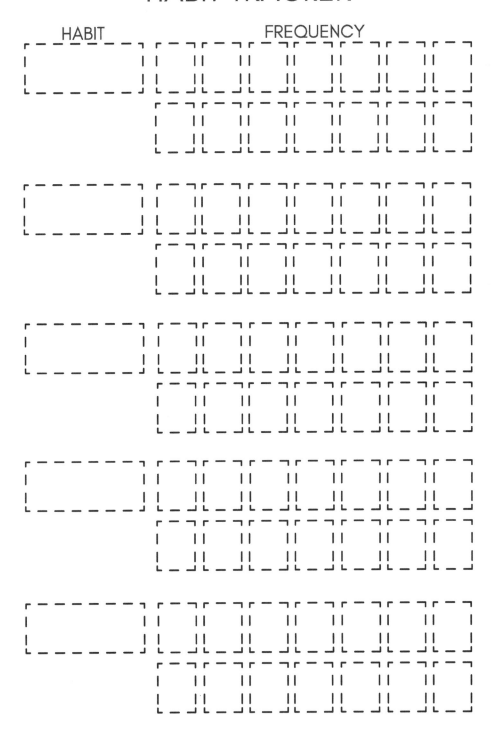

FOOD	QUANTITY	CALORIES/VALUE
		TOTAL

FOOD	QUANTITY	CALORIES/VALUE
		TOTAL

EXERCISE LOG

DATE	ACTIVITY	DURATION

MOOD TRACKER

GIVE A COLOUR TO EACH MOOD AND
COLOUR IN YOUR MOOD AT THE END
OF EACH DAY TO KEEP TRACK

HAPPY

STRESSED

SAD

NEUTRAL

FOCUSED

CALM

M   T   W   T   F   S   S

HABIT TRACKER

HABIT   FREQUENCY

FOOD	QUANTITY	CALORIES/VALUE
		TOTAL

FOOD	QUANTITY	CALORIES/VALUE
		TOTAL

FOOD	QUANTITY	CALORIES/VALUE
		TOTAL

FOOD	QUANTITY	CALORIES/VALUE
		TOTAL

FOOD	QUANTITY	CALORIES/VALUE
		TOTAL

FOOD	QUANTITY	CALORIES/VALUE
		TOTAL

HABIT TRACKER

HABIT   FREQUENCY

MOOD TRACKER

GIVE A COLOUR TO EACH MOOD AND
COLOUR IN YOUR MOOD AT THE END
OF EACH DAY TO KEEP TRACK

HAPPY

STRESSED

SAD

NEUTRAL

FOCUSED

CALM

M   T   W   T   F   S   S

EXERCISE LOG

DATE	ACTIVITY	DURATION

FOOD	QUANTITY	CALORIES/VALUE
		TOTAL

FOOD	QUANTITY	CALORIES/VALUE
		TOTAL

FOOD	QUANTITY	CALORIES/VALUE
		TOTAL

FOOD	QUANTITY	CALORIES/VALUE
		TOTAL

FOOD	QUANTITY	CALORIES/VALUE
		TOTAL

FOOD	QUANTITY	CALORIES/VALUE
		TOTAL

FOOD	QUANTITY	CALORIES/VALUE
		TOTAL

MOOD TRACKER

GIVE A COLOUR TO EACH MOOD AND
COLOUR IN YOUR MOOD AT THE END
OF EACH DAY TO KEEP TRACK

HAPPY

STRESSED

SAD

NEUTRAL

FOCUSED

CALM

M   T   W   T   F   S   S

EXERCISE LOG

DATE	ACTIVITY	DURATION

HABIT TRACKER

HABIT

FREQUENCY

Printed in Great Britain
by Amazon